Coconut Oil Skin and Hair Care Guide: How to Use Coconut Oil for Healthy and Beautiful Skin and Hair

by R. Johnson

Disclaimer:

This information is provided for consumer informational and educational purposes only and may not reflect the most current information available. This book is sold with the understanding the author and/or publisher is not giving medical advice, nor should the information contained in this book replace medical advice, nor is it intended to diagnose or treat any disease, illness or other medical condition. Always consult your medical practitioner before making any dietary changes or treating or attempting to treat any medical condition. Do not disregard, avoid, or delay seeking medical advice because of something you may have read in this book.

While we endeavor to keep the information up to date and correct, we make no representations or warranties of any kind, express or implied, about the completeness, accuracy, reliability, suitability or availability with respect to the book or the information, products, services, or related graphics contained book for any purpose. Any reliance you place on such information is therefore strictly at your own risk.

Dedication:

This book is dedicated to all those who have discovered the many benefits of coconut oil. Keep up the good work. This book wouldn't have been possible without the pioneers who have tried coconut oil on anything and everything skin- and health-related.

Contents

Coconut Oil: What Is It?

Coconut oil is oil extracted from the meat of coconuts. While it's technically an oil, it's a white solid when the ambient room temperature is below 76 degrees F. As the temperature creeps above 76 degrees, the oil melts into a clear or yellow-tinted liquid.

It's edible, and there are a number of health benefits associated with eating it, but that isn't what this book is all about. In addition to being a healthy dietary supplement, coconut oil is great for your skin and hair. It contains a number of fatty acids, including capric acid, caprylic acid and lauric acid, which have the following therapeutic properties:

- Antibacterial.
- Antifungal.
- Antimicrobial.
- Antioxidant.

What this means is coconut oil is able to kill unhealthy bacteria, fungi and microorganisms on contact. It's able to fight off infections and can be used to prevent oxidative stress placed on the body by reactive oxygen and free radicals. The medium chain triglycerides in coconut oil are able to penetrate deep within the skin, where they get right to work eliminating toxins and rendering harmful microorganisms inactive.

While there are health experts that advise against consumption of coconut oil because of its high saturated fat content, you'd be hard-pressed to find a skin or hair care expert who recommends against using coconut oil on the skin. In fact, a number of the most beautiful men and women in the world swear by coconut oil as one of their go-to products for healthy looking skin and hair. They know what you're about to learn. Coconut oil has moisturizing and regenerative qualities and can be used to rejuvenate and revitalize skin and hair that's been damaged by years of abuse.

Coconut oil can be used on its own or it can be used as a base oil for a number of skin and hair care products. Massage therapists blend it with other oils and butters and massage it into the muscles of their clients. It's also used in a number of soaps, creams, salves and tonics. Aromatherapists combine it with essential oils to dilute them to the point where they won't irritate the skin upon contact. Soap makers also sometimes use coconut oil as the fat they need for the saponification process, which is the process in which lye is transformed into soap.

There are many, many ways coconut oil can be used to improve your health. While numerous books have been written on the benefits of consuming coconut oil, there aren't many books solely dedicated to the many benefits of applying coconut oil topically. Topical application of coconut oil is usually relegated to a small section in most books and is more of an afterthought than anything. If you're interested in coconut oil and how it can be applied to your skin and hair, this is the book for you.

The best part about coconut oil is it's completely natural. Buy the right type of oil and you're applying something that's devoid of the nasty and harsh chemicals found in most beauty products sold in stores today. Instead of slowly poisoning yourself with chemicals, make the switch to coconut oil and get started down the path to recovery.

Your body will thank you for it and your skin and hair will be healthier as a result.

There's Only One Type of Coconut Oil You Should Use

Most stores only stock small jars of a brand or two of coconut oil and it tends to be rather expensive. Looking at store shelves, you'd think coconut oil was a specialty item that nobody buys. Unless you have a good health food store or a Costco near you that carries coconut oil at a decent price, you're much better off ordering coconut oil online. Type "coconut oil" into a search engine and you're presented with hundreds of choices. There are multiple brands and a variety of types of coconut oil. Pressed, refined, virgin, organic. It's enough to make your head spin. Prices vary widely, even amongst similar types of oil, which can further confuse things when trying to choose the right oil.

I'm going to make things very easy on you by telling you there's only one type of coconut oil you should use.

All you need to have on-hand is organic virgin cold-pressed coconut oil. It's the best of best, free of chemicals and processed in the manner that helps the oil retain the highest level of beneficial components during the minimal processing it undergoes. The rest of the chapter is going to be spent discussing what cold-pressed virgin coconut oil is and why it's preferable to the other types. It's good information to have, but isn't absolutely necessary for you to know. You can skip ahead to the next chapter if you'd like to get right into the benefits of using coconut oil.

The rest of the book assumes you're using virgin cold-pressed coconut oil. Going organic isn't absolutely necessary, but there are some definite benefits, as we'll discuss later in this chapter. Remember, every time you see coconut oil mentioned later in the book, if a type of coconut oil isn't specified, it's cold-pressed virgin coconut oil I'm referring to.

Extraction Methods

Coconut oil comes from the meat of the coconut. In order to get coconut oil, the oil has to be *extracted*, or removed, from the meat. As with anything that has to be extracted, people are ingenious and have come up with a number of ways to extract coconut oil. Since the medium chain fatty acids found in coconut oil are easily damaged by heat, the extraction method used to draw the oil from the meat largely determines the quality of the final product. The more heat that is used, the lower the quality of the oil.

Cold-pressed oil is extracted by either pressing or grinding the meat of the coconut to extract the oil without raising the temperature above 120 degrees F. This allows the oil to retain its original flavor, while maintaining its natural nutrient level and aroma. Since excess heat isn't created during the extraction process, the oil retains its chemical structure and remains recognizable to the body.

Expeller-pressed oil is extracted using a machine that screws down and presses the oil from the coconut meat. The biggest difference between expeller-pressed and cold-pressed oils is the amount of heat produced by the pressing process. Expeller-pressing can heat the oil up to more than 200 degrees F, which can destroy the structure of the fatty acids, causing them to turn into trans fats. It can also cause harmful free radicals to form, which aren't something you want to put on your skin or into your body.

The *centrifuge method* of extraction also heats the oil up, albeit to a lesser extent. With this method, coconut meat is placed into a *centrifuge*, which is a large machine that spins the meat in circles at a high rate of speed to separate the oil from the meat. While the risk of trans fat formation and oxidation isn't as high as with expeller-pressed oils, water is mixed in with the coconut oil during the extraction process, which makes the oil more likely to go rancid.

Chemical extraction uses toxic chemicals to draw the oil out of the coconut. Chemicals can be used on their own or combined with one of the other methods. Chemical solvents like hexane are often used to dissolve the coconut, making it easier for the oil to be withdrawn. The hexane is separated from the oil at a later step, but trace amounts of the chemical are left behind. Chemically-extracted oils are the worst of the bunch and shouldn't be used for topical application or consumption.

When it comes to extraction methods, choose cold-pressed oils and you won't be sorry. You'll be getting chemical-free oil extracted using a process that generates the least amount of heat and in doing so does the least amount of damage to the structure of the oil.

People often ask how they can tell what extraction method is used to obtain the coconut oil they're buying. What I've found is the expeller-pressed and cold-pressed oils are usually labeled as such on the label. These are the manufacturing methods preferred by most consumers, so the manufacturers clearly label their containers when these methods are used. The other methods of extraction aren't usually on the labels, at least not on any I've seen. You probably won't ever see "Hexane-extracted" on a coconut oil label because nobody would buy it.

If you have a brand of coconut oil you like and the extraction method isn't specifically named on the label, get on the phone and call the manufacturer. They'll usually be willing to tell you how the oil is extracted. If you find out chemicals are used in the process, it's time to find a healthier alternative.

Virgin vs. Refined

Most coconut oil is made from *copra*, which is the dried meat of the coconut. Copra is dried using a number of methods, including kiln drying, sun drying and smoke drying. The copra drying process can contaminate the meat with poly-aromatic hydrocarbons and the oil that's extracted from it isn't pure.

Copra is often shipped over long distances in large amounts to the factories where coconut oil is produced. Unsanitary conditions during shipping and storage can create an environment in which toxins can contaminate the copra and the oil made from the copra. When coconut oil is processed from copra, it has to undergo heavy processing to eliminate the toxins and to make it fit for human consumption.

The refinement process involves at least three steps and can involve many more. High heat is used to remove the coconut scent and flavor from the oil and chemicals or bleaching clays are used to bleach the oil. Chemical solvents are sometimes used in the extraction process and the refined coconut oil is sometimes partially-hydrogenated, which is a process that transforms unsaturated fats into saturated fats, leaving trans fats in its wake. Sodium hydroxide is often added to increase the amount of time the oil can be left sitting on the shelf.

Virgin or extra-virgin coconut oil is oil that hasn't gone through the refinement process. It's pure oil that's been extracted from wet coconut meat or meat that's undergone a drying process that doesn't contaminate the meat. The oil is typically extracted within a day of the coconuts being harvested, so there's little chance of the coconut meat going bad.

The oil is pure when it is extracted and doesn't have to be highly processed to make it fit for consumption. It isn't exposed to the high heat, chemicals and bleaching process refined oils go through, so it retains both the coconut flavor and the aroma of the coconut it came from.

Virgin coconut oil is often labeled as "extra-virgin" oil. There is no set of standards that separate oil labeled as "virgin" from oil labeled as "extra-virgin," so be aware that you probably aren't going to get better oil by paying more for extra-virgin oil. Find a reputable supplier and don't worry about whether the label says "extra-virgin" or "virgin." It's more of a marketing ploy than anything. You're much better off looking into the manufacturing methods used to make the oil when trying to determine whether a certain brand of oil is right for you.

Organic Coconut Oil

Organic oils are derived from organically-grown coconut crops. This means no chemicals have been sprayed on the trees during the growing process. No herbicides or pesticides are sprayed on the trees and no chemicals are used on the coconuts, the meat or the oil after harvesting. The coconuts harvested won't contain the same levels of chemicals, pesticides and herbicides found in traditional crops.

If you can't find organic coconut oil, don't let that stop you. Studies have shown the levels of pesticides found in coconut oil to be extremely low. If it's available, it's marginally safer, but don't let that be the reason you don't purchase coconut oil.

There's another good reason to go organic that doesn't have to do with the health benefits it affords you. It has to do with the overall health of the planet.

When you buy organic, you get the added benefit of knowing you're buying coconut oil made from coconuts that have been sustainably grown and harvested. Organic farmers are usually more in tune with the environment because they can't simply add more chemicals to the ground when things start to go wrong. They don't pump their soil full of chemicals that are then allowed to run off into nearby lakes, rivers and aquifers. The people working on organic farms are healthier because they aren't forced to work in close proximity to toxic herbicides and fertilizers.

The price difference between coconut oil made from organic and traditionally-grown coconuts is negligible and you can find organic oil for around the same price as regular oil, especially when you get into the larger-sized containers. There's no good reason not to buy organic coconut oil, especially when you consider the growing practices used with traditional crops.

Why Coconut Oil Is So Good for Your Skin

Healthy skin often equates to a happy and healthy life. When a person's skin looks radiant, they feel better and are more confident way. Unhealthy skin can have the opposite effect, leaving a person with a low sense of self-worth that bleeds into other areas of life. Poor skin doesn't just impact life at home, it can affect a person to the point that it can be detrimental in all areas of that person's life, from work to personal life and everything in between.

For this reason, people are often willing to spend large sums of money on the latest and greatest specialty creams concocted by laboratories looking to milk them for every last dime they have. These creams sometimes work, but more often than not fall far short of the mark. People pay the steep prices manufacturers are asking for them, but they rarely, if ever, get what they want from them. Anti-aging creams, lotions, salves, you name it. All are designed and marketed to get you to open your wallet. The more money spent on research and development, the more you're going to end up paying.

Read the label attached to these creams, salves and tonics and you'll more often than not find a list of synthetic chemicals that have been cooked up by scientists to "solve" problems. These chemicals are rarely beneficial and many are known to cause problems when applied in large amounts. Don't assume just because something's sold in stores that it's completely safe. While there are restrictions as to what can be included in skin care products, manufacturers are afforded a lot of leeway.

It helps to remember that any cream you rub into your skin is going to be absorbed into your body. The tiny capillaries that lay just under your skin take up the chemicals and distribute them across your body via your bloodstream. Once inside, they aren't going to do you any good. Even if they aren't problematic (and some are), the body has to waste valuable resources clearing itself of them. One or two uses probably won't cause issues, but the accumulated damage done through repeated application might result in health problems years down the road—and you may not ever associate the problems you're having then with the skin care product you're using now.

Since skin creams make their way inside the body and into the blood stream, it's important to use natural products the body can recognize, products that the body knows and welcomes because they're natural and healthy. This is where coconut oil really comes into its own. Coconut oil is as close to a one-stop natural remedy for skin problems as you can get. It works on all sorts of skin problems and is able to be used by people with most skin types. Wrinkles, dry skin, oily skin and acne are just a handful of the problems coconut oil is believed to be able to help.

Coconut oil has the following beneficial qualities that make it a great all-purpose skin cream and one that can be used as a home remedy for a number of skin problems:

- Coconut oil has been shown to be antibacterial, antifungal, antiviral and antioxidant by nature.
- Coconut oil is antimicrobial and kills harmful microbes on contact.
- It can be used as a base oil or carrier oil in the creation of oil blends that have even more therapeutic qualities.
- It helps the skin heal and regenerate.
- It helps the skin retain moisture and improves hydration.
- It provides a protective barrier between the skin and the air.
- It relieves dryness and itching.
- It's all-natural and doesn't contain harmful synthetic chemicals.
- The fats in coconut oil act as an emollient and soften the skin by increasing the levels of surface lipids.
- The medium chain triglycerides in coconut oil provide nutrition to the skin and the cells beneath the skin.

Coconut oil does all this and more.

You'd be hard-pressed to find another cream or salve, man-made or not that can claim all these benefits—unless it has coconut oil in it. You can take care of a number of skin-related issues and possibly stop aging dead in its tracks through use of coconut oil. People the world over are realizing the benefits and coconut oil is rapidly gaining in popularity, both as a skin care product and as a dietary supplement.

In fact, coconut oil works best for the skin when it's used both internally and externally at the same time. It can be used to fight topical infections at the point of infection, while it fights inflammation and helps prevent the infection from spreading internally.

Coconut Oil as a Carrier Oil

While there are definite benefits to using coconut oil on its own, it can also be used as a *carrier oil*, which is oil used to dilute and deliver essential oils to the skin. Essential oils are the powerful essences of plants and are often too strong to be applied directly to the skin. Using a carrier oil like coconut oil allows you to take the strength of an essential oil or blend of oils down a few notches to the point where it can be applied to the skin and massaged into it with little worry of irritation.

Essential oils and other concentrated oils can cause severe irritation when applied directly to the skin. The reaction can be a minor one, in which the user suffers minor redness and inflammation, or it can be a major allergic reaction. Certain oils are considered "hotter" than others and have to be diluted heavily before application. Do your due diligence before using essential oils because what you don't know could hurt you. Some oils are so hot they should never be applied to the skin, diluted or not.

Interesting oil blends can be created where you mix various vegetable oils and essential oils to create blends with interesting scents and varying therapeutic benefits. There are literally hundreds of thousands of blends you can create that smell great and will benefit your health in a number of ways. If you aren't sure where to start, enlist the help of an aromatherapy specialist or read up on how to use essential oils to your benefit. There is a ton of good information out there, including my book, *The Aromatherapy and Essential Oils Handbook*.

Yes, that was just a shameless self-promotion of one of my other books. Here's a link to it if you're interested:

http://www.amazon.com/dp/B00BECCJXY

When using coconut oil to dilute essential oils, always start off by mixing small amounts of the essential oil into large amounts of coconut oil. Test your skin's tolerance of the oil using tiny amounts of oil mixed into liberal amounts of coconut oil.

Mix a drop or two of your chosen essential oil into a couple tablespoons of coconut oil and test it by applying it to a small patch of skin in an inconspicuous area. Wait for at least 12 hours to see if there's a reaction. Whenever you try a new oil or oil blend, always be sure to test it using small amounts of the essential oils you're using. If you have a reaction to a diluted blend, you know you aren't going to be able to use the blend at full strength. If you do have a reaction to a certain essential oil, try applying coconut oil or another vegetable oil to the affected area. It may help to further dilute the essential oil and ease the reaction. If the reaction is severe, seek immediate medical care. Severe reactions to essential oils are rare, but they can take place.

Virgin coconut oil has a coconut scent that must be taken into consideration when creating aromatic blends. Stronger essential oils will overpower the coconut scent, but the coconut scent will mix with lighter scents. Exotic and interesting aromas can be created when mixing coconut oil with essential oils. Some aromatherapists recommend using *fractionated coconut oil*, which doesn't have the same coconut scent and is a lighter oil, but you lose a lot of the health benefits of coconut oil when you switch to fractionated oil. Fractionated oil is altered oil and isn't coconut oil in its purest form, so it's avoided by those looking to use only pure oils.

Aromatherapy can be beneficial in a number of ways, but there are a number of pitfalls and problems a rookie can encounter. It can help to enlist the help of an aromatherapy professional, especially in the beginning when you're just learning the ropes. You're going to have questions—and they're best answered by someone who's been there and done that.

The Skin as an Organ

Ask someone to name an organ and they'll more than likely answer with an internal organ like the heart, the lungs or the liver. While we may not think of the skin on our bodies as an organ, the skin is the largest organ found on the human body. It's a living, breathing system of cells, nerves and capillaries that combine to cover the entire outside of the human body. Skin is designed to keep the good stuff in and the bad stuff out.

The skin is tasked with insulating the body from the outside world. It helps shield the body against heat and cold, it protects you from the harmful rays emitted by the sun and it prevents harmful microorganisms from gaining easy access into the body. It's like a giant shield, wrapped around your body to keep everything inside in good working order.

In addition to protects the inner workings of the body, the skin acts as the body's interface with the outside world. It's packed with nerve endings that sense the smallest changes in conditions on the outside and relay them to your brain. The skin is the reason you know when it's too cold or too hot and are able to react to the changes before you freeze to death or burn up. Without the skin and its many nerve endings, you could do irreparable damage to your body without even realizing it. Without the sensory input of the skin, you could unknowingly back up into a hot fire and not know it until you smelled the burning flesh. By then the damage would be severe—and possibly irreparable.

Your skin is responsible for the following tasks:

- Fighting off infections.
- Healing itself when injured.
- Sensing when you touch or brush up against things.
- Keeping harmful bacteria out.
- Preventing blood and water from evaporating from your body.
- Protecting the body from heat, cold and light.
- Regulating the temperature of your body.
- Sensing when microorganisms are trying to enter and ringing the alarm.
- Storing fat and water.

The thickness and characteristics of your skin vary depending on where on your body it's found. Some areas of skin, like your head and pubic area, have numerous follicles that grow hair. Other areas, like your palms and the soles of your feet, are largely devoid of hair follicles. The skin is much thicker in these areas than it is around the rest of the body. This is because these are the most-used parts of your body and they endure the most abuse. Millions of years of evolution have thickened the skin in these areas because you need it to be thick to withstand the amount of use your hands and feet see on a daily basis.

No matter where on your body the skin is found, it is made up of three basic layers: the subcutaneous layer, the dermis and the epidermis. The *subcutaneous layer* is the base layer and it's made up of collagen and fat cells. These cells keep the body warm by keeping heat from leaking out and they act as an impact shield when the body takes a hard blow.

The *dermis* is the middle layer. It's sandwiched between the subcutaneous layer and the epidermis. This is the layer of skin that contains the sweat glands, blood vessels, lymph vessels, hair follicles and the nerves. It's all glued together by *collagen*, which is the material that gives the skin strength and allows it to flex and bend. It's also the layer of skin that's responsible for wrinkles, which form as the collagen in the skin becomes weak and begins to break down.

The outer layer of the skin is the *epidermis*. It's made of three interrelated layers. The base layer is the *basal layer*. It contains *basal cells*, which are highly active cells that continuously divide to form new cells called *keratinocytes*. The keratinocytes form the *squamous cell layer*, which is made of live keratinocytes. As the keratinocytes age, they move up to the top layer of the epidermis, the *stratum corneum*, also known as the horny layer. As the keratinocytes die, they are shed from the skin in a continuous cycle. It's this outer layer of skin that's responsible for keeping harmful organisms from entering the body. A break in this layer can let all sorts of harmful stuff in.

Skin Disorders

Because it's on the outside instead of being on the inside like most organs, the skin is one of the most vulnerable organs of the human body. Luckily, it's also one of the most durable, because it can fall victim to a number of ailments and disorders that, while rarely life threatening, can cause discomfort and irritation. Breaks in the skin can lead to *systemic infections*, or infections that make their way throughout the body once they find an opening through which they're able to enter.

In addition to the physical damage done to the skin, many skin disorders also do psychological damage because they're visible and they cause the sufferer extreme stress.

The following skin disorders afflict millions of people worldwide. They run the gamut from mildly irritating to downright life-altering and many can be debilitative in nature if allowed to get bad enough. The following skin disorders are impacting lives across the nation as we speak:

- Acne.
- Dry skin.
- Infections.
- Inflammation.
- Psoriasis.
- Rosacea.
- Scars.

Coconut oil can be used to alleviate the effects of all of the items on the list. The next several chapters cover how to best use coconut oil when you have some of these issues.

Acne

Acne, known in the medical world as *acne vulgaris* in its most common form, is the number one most common skin problem in the world today. You'd be hard-pressed to find a person, man or woman, who has made it to adulthood with nary a pimple. For some, acne is a minor bump in the road during puberty and all but disappears by the time adulthood rolls around. For others, acne is the bane of their existence.

This skin disease occurs when the sebaceous glands in the skin become clogged and can no longer release sebum. When they become plugged with oil and dead skin cells (and other stuff), irritation occurs, leading to the red mound most of us know all too well. That's right, I'm talking about the dreaded pimple. They most commonly occur on the face, but can be found pretty much anywhere on the body, with the head, neck, chest and back being the most common places for them to occur. Acne can run the gamut from mild to severe, with the most severe cases being characterized by certain areas of the body appearing to be covered in large painful pimples.

When excess sebum clogs hair follicles, *comedones* are formed. This is a fancy term to describe whiteheads and blackheads as a group. The backed-up follicles create an environment in which bacteria can thrive and the bacteria levels start to climb. If the pressure of the buildup causes the follicle wall to rupture, sebum begins to leak out into the nearby tissue. Inflammation occurs and you get a raised pustule.

There is no single cure for acne.

This is largely because there isn't a single cause of acne. Instead, it's caused by a number of factors that all combine to create conditions conducive to acne forming. Those with overly active oil glands and oily skin tend to be more prone to acne, as are those whose skin produces dead skin cells at a faster rate than others. When the skin doesn't shed dead cells at a fast enough rate, acne can occur if the skin cells accumulate to the point that they start clogging pores. Hormonal imbalances and stress levels can also affect whether or not a person is prone to acne.

Can Coconut Oil Provide Acne Relief?

Coconut oil has been touted by some as a miracle cure for acne. There are seemingly people everywhere who use and espouse its many virtues when it comes to acne relief. One thing's for certain . . . There are a lot of people who swear by it. This begs the question of whether or not it's as good as people say.

The answer is a solid maybe. For some, it works wonders. For other, maybe not so much.

It has definite acne fighting qualities that work in a similar manner to some of the more prevalent acne medications in use today. Most acne experts recommend treating acne with topical applications of benzoyl peroxide. This is the active ingredient in many over the counter and prescription acne medications. It works by killing the bacteria causing the infections that cause acne. No bacterial overgrowth equals no inflamed pimples to make you wish you could hide in your room forever—or at least until the pimple fades away. The reason benzoyl peroxide works so well is because it has strong antimicrobial properties.

Benzoyl peroxide tends to be a bit harsh and can dry out the skin of those who use products containing it, especially those using extra-strength products. If you've ever rubbed acne medication into your skin and wondered why your skin felt taut or tight right after use, you've felt benzoyl peroxide at work. This effect is worse for some than it is for others.

Coconut oil has similar, albeit slightly weaker, antimicrobial properties as benzoyl peroxide. The lauric and capric acid found in coconut oil are both antimicrobial by nature. This is a bit of a double-edged sword. On one hand, using coconut oil won't give you the same bang for your buck as benzoyl peroxide when it comes to killing off bacteria. On the other hand, it may work well for those with sensitive skin that dries out quickly when benzoyl peroxide is used.

In addition to killing off acne-causing bacteria, the anti-inflammatory properties of coconut oil can help knock down the swelling associated with existing acne. Pimples don't disappear immediately upon contact, but they will be less severe and of a shorter duration than they normally would.

While many acne treatments damage the skin and cause new problems to crop up, coconut oil is beneficial in that it strengthens and moisturizes the skin. It's all-natural and doesn't use harsh chemicals to kill the bacteria that causes acne. Instead, it contains natural antimicrobial agents that act in a gentler manner.

While coconut oil does have some qualities that make it a good acne fighting remedy for some, it does have its downside. While the reason behind it isn't entirely understood, some people see their acne start to clear up when they first start using coconut oil, only to have it return with a vengeance. This may be part of the body's cleansing process and some people have indeed found they can continue using coconut oil and the new breakout will clear up and their skin will start to clear. Once the impurities have been drawn out of the skin, the new acne flare-up sometimes clears up. Others have to stop using coconut oil entirely, as their breakouts either worsen or stay the same over time and don't get any better.

There's a lot of speculation out there that coconut oil clogs the pores of the skin, causing more problems than it solves. For a select few, this appears to be the case, but this isn't the case with everyone. Coconut oil appears to be a slightly *comodegenic* substance, meaning it can cause problems in people who are highly susceptible to clogged pores, but it doesn't have the same effect on everyone. What this means is the antibacterial effects of coconut oil may help some people, but this effect may be outweighed by the comodegenic effect the oil has in people who are highly susceptible to getting clogged pores.

The answer to the question of whether coconut oil is a miracle cure for acne is a resounding maybe. If you're one of the lucky people who it works for, then coconut oil can be a great natural remedy. On the other hand, if you're one of the unlucky few who experiences worse breakouts as a result of using coconut oil, then it's anything but helpful. The only way to find out for sure is to try it and see, preferably in an inconspicuous area where a new breakout won't be too obvious.

Discuss coconut oil with your doctor before using it in an acne prone area to see if he or she thinks it's worth a shot. If so, try it in a small area first to see what happens. And remember, more isn't always better, especially when it comes to oils you're rubbing into your skin. It should be used in small amounts instead of being slathered all over your face and body. If your acne gets a lot worse, then discontinue use. If it gets better in the small area, then consider expanding the area you're using it on. Just be aware that the reaction isn't always immediate. Some former users of coconut oil indicate their acne didn't start to get worse until a week or two after they started using it. Be aware it can also take a while for acne to start clearing up.

Using Coconut Oil for Acne

Most people use coconut oil as a standalone agent when they use it for acne. Applying it topically twice a day in small amounts is usually sufficient. The face should be thoroughly cleaned before application for best results. Most people apply it in the morning when they wake up and at night when they go to bed. For severe acne, it may need to be applied more frequently. Some literature recommends applying it 3 to 4 times a day when acne is prevalent.

Those not prone to clogged pores can apply it topically and rub it into the skin and leave it on, as one would a cream or a salve. This will give the coconut oil time to really work its way into the pores where it'll start killing off the bacteria that cause acne infections. It nourishes the skin and is thought to help unclog already clogged pores while removing impurities from the skin. An initial acne flare-up isn't always a bad thing, as it can be indicative of impurities being drawn from the skin. If the flare-up doesn't begin to improve within a week, discontinue use of coconut oil.

Because of its anti-inflammatory properties, coconut oil can also be used as a spot-treatment for individual pimples. Simply apply a bit of coconut oil to a stubborn pimple and wait. The inflammation should subside quickly and the pimple will fade away. Don't pop pimples you plan on treating in this manner. It will take longer for the irritation caused by popping the pimple to go away and scar tissue can form. The pimple will fade away, but a nasty scar can be left behind.

Speaking of acne scarring, coconut oil can be used to help fade scars away as well. The nutrients found in coconut oil promote the healing of damaged skin, which can help scarring fade away at a faster rate than normal. It may not have much effect on deep scarring, but minor scars will fade away quickly.

In addition to applying coconut oil topically to help with acne, it can also be ingested. It helps balance the body and can act on acne from both the inside and out. Coconut oil helps detoxify the liver and aids the body in maintaining a healthy balance of beneficial bacteria in the gut. A teaspoon or two of coconut oil taken daily as a supplement can also help ease the inflammation associated with acne, as well as helping level out the hormone imbalance often associated with excess sebum production.

Essential Oils

Another way coconut oil can be used for acne is to use it as a carrier oil for essential oils that are known to be beneficial to those who are suffering from acne. Essential oils can be effective at killing acne bacteria and easing inflammation, so you get a potent one-two punch when you combine coconut oil with essential oils. Combine an antibacterial oil with one that's known for toning the skin and closing up the pores and you've got an effective oil blend that doesn't just kill bacteria—it prevents new pimples from forming by locking the pores down so oil won't build up in them.

While most essential oils are antibacterial in nature, many of them are too strong to be applied topically, even when diluted in coconut oil or another carrier oil. They can burn the skin and have been known to cause severe allergic reactions that sensitize the skin to the point where essential oils can no longer be used without causing a similar reaction.

The following essential oils have strong antibacterial properties and can be used to fight acne:

- **Lavender.** This gentle oil is one of the few essential oils that people are able to apply at full strength with little risk of adverse reaction. It's antibacterial and anti-inflammatory and is a good choice for most people. It's also effective at helping fade scarring due to acne.
- **Tea tree.** It's stronger than lavender, but is still gentle enough to be able to be used in conjunction with coconut oil by most people. Tea tree oil is strongly antimicrobial and is widely considered one of the best essential oils for acne.
- **Bergamot.** Bergamot oil is antiseptic and astringent by nature. It works well for those with oily skin, but should be avoided by people who already suffer from dry skin.
- **Lemongrass.** This astringent oil is another oil that works good for those who suffer from oily skin. It's antimicrobial and antibacterial and is a natural astringent.
- **Clove oil.** This oil is extremely strong and should be highly diluted before use. It works

well to kill acne-causing bacteria, but isn't a good choice for those with overly sensitive skin because of its strength. Try diluting it in a mixture of Grapeseed and coconut oil for best results.

To use essential oils in conjunction with coconut oil as an acne remedy, combine few drops of your favorite oil or oils with a teaspoon of coconut oil and stir them in. Apply the oil blend topically and massage it into the skin. Always test new oil blends on a small patch of skin first and watch for a reaction. If a reaction occurs, discontinue use of the oil blend immediately.

Turmeric

Turmeric, a pungent Indian spice typically using in the culinary world, can be combined with coconut oil and applied to the skin as a homemade acne cream. In India, turmeric has been in use for hundreds of years, not just for food, but for application to the skin to cure a number of skin problems. It contains a chemical compound called *curcumin*, which has been shown in at least one recent study to fight the main bacteria responsible for inflammatory acne. Curcumin builds up in the skin and effectively blocks propionibacterium acnes from building up.

Curcumin needs a lipid to deliver it into the skin. The study used lauric acid, which is found in abundance in coconut oil. It stands to reason that coconut oil could be combined with turmeric to create a homemade cream that would be effective in treating acne because it's packed with compounds that both kill harmful bacteria and prevent the growth of new bacteria.

Using turmeric can stain the skin a light yellow color. Regular turmeric is known for staining the skin, so try to find "katsuri" turmeric, which some say is less likely to stain. Use turmeric in small amounts and use it at night, so you can wash it off with soap and warm water in the morning.

Skin Infections

Since your skin is the barrier between your body and germs, it comes in contact with a lot of nasty stuff. Viruses, bacteria, fungi and parasites all make their way onto your skin on a daily basis. For the most part, your skin does a good job of protecting you from microbial infections and germs.

Most of the time, you won't even know when your skin has repelled a pathogen. It happens more often than you'd probably like to know. Most of the time it happens without your body skipping a beat because the pathogens never make it past the skin.

On occasion, your skin may react to one of these agents, either because it is attempting to enter the body through a break in the skin or it begins attacking the body through the skin. When this takes place, infection can occur. The virus, bacteria or fungi attempts to enter the body, provoking the body to respond by attacking the virus. This is a natural response that often takes place behind the scenes without you ever knowing it. You may not feel it all, or you could suffer side effects you never associate with your body fighting an infection.

The immune system of the host can often fight off infection on its own. *Acute infections* are relatively short-term infections that the body takes care of on its own, often without the host realizing he or she has been infected. Other times, general symptoms may appear, but they may not be immediately linked to an infection. They come and go as the body fights off the infection, with the host none the wiser.

When a pathogen gets past the outer layer of the skin, the body's immune system takes over the fight to protect your body against the invader. Special blood cells are sent out on a mission to hunt down the source of the infection and kill it. Special white blood cells called *neutrophils* flood the area where the infection is trying to take hold. They take the fight right to the point of infection and attempt to kill or inactivate the agent causing the infection.

Coconut oil can help fight off both bacterial and fungal infections. Let's take a closer look at each of these types of infections.

The Use of Coconut Oil on Bacterial Infections

Bacterial infections tend to be rather nasty infections because bacteria start releasing toxins once they've taken hold inside the body. This type of infection is caused by bad bacteria that begin to wreak havoc once they enter the body. It's important to note not all bacteria are bad. It's estimated that less than one percent of all bacteria are bad bacteria. The rest are either neutral or are beneficial to the body in some way.

The normal course of treatment for a bacterial infection involves using strong antibiotics to knock down the infection by killing off the bacteria causing it. Many of these antibiotics don't target the bacteria you want to kill. Instead, they kill off many beneficial bacteria along with the harmful bacteria you actually want gone. This can throw off the balance of good bacteria in your body, which can lead to the bacteria you're trying to get rid of or other harmful bacteria being able to regrow after you stop taking the antibiotics—and this time there aren't any other bacteria to compete with them. This can lead to a worse infection that's even harder to get rid of the second time around.

Another downside to antibiotics is the proclivity of bacteria to build up a resistance to them. The more antibiotics you take, the more likely you are to create a resistance to those antibiotics. You may create a bacterial strain that can't easily be cured by antibiotics and since bacterial infections can often be passed to others, they may struggle to clear their infections up as well. When *superbacteria* form, antibiotics won't work well or won't work at all, and by using them, you'll help the bacteria grow even more resistant. While antibiotics may be necessary for the worst infections, they're often the first thing people turn to for minor issues that could be taken care of through natural and less invasive treatments.

The strong antibacterial and anti-inflammatory properties of coconut oil make it a good natural solution for a number of bacterial infections. Since it's all-natural, the bacteria you're killing don't build up an immunity to it. Coconut oil can be used repeatedly on pathogens with little risk of them building immunity. It can be used in conjunction with and sometimes instead of antibiotics to knock down infections.

Some bacterial infections can be life-threatening if allowed to blossom out of control, so always consult with your doctor before attempting to use coconut oil to rid yourself of a bacterial infection. There may be underlying medical concerns or reasons you shouldn't use coconut oil.

Staph Infections

Staph infections are highly contagious and potentially dangerous skin infections caused by any one of 30 different Staphylococcus bacteria. *Staphlyococcus aureus* is the most common and is the cause of most staph infections. Anyone can get a staph infection and all it takes is coming into contact with the bacteria when you have a break in your skin into which the bacteria can creep.

This sort of infection can range from anything from a minor superficial infection that's irritating, but isn't overly dangerous, to a painful and potentially life-threatening infection that could end in the loss of both life and limb.

While staph infections of the skin can be bad, even worse things can happen when staph bacteria gets into the blood stream. Pneumonia, blood poisoning and toxic shock syndrome can all come about as a result of a staph infection.

When staph infections present themselves as a skin infection, they often start off looking innocent enough. A red mark here, a red bump there. Then, seemingly out of nowhere, they take off. Boils, pimples, redness, swelling and pain are all common symptoms. Inflammation kicks in as the body tries to fight the infection and pus and other fluids may start draining from the infected area. Staph infections can be red and swollen and can leave nasty scarring behind once they go away. *Cellulitis*, which is a deeper skin infection characterized by even more swelling and pain, can occur.

Methicillin-resistant Staphylococcus aureus (MSRA) is a particularly persistent type of staph infection that's resistant to certain antibiotics. It's difficult to treat because normal treatments often won't work against this pathogen. MSRA not only affects the skin, it also poisons the body by releasing toxins into the bloodstream.

Coconut oil has been shown to inactive the MSRA virus and can be an effective tool in protecting the body against certain other staph infections. When applied topically, coconut oil inactivates the virus before it can get into the skin. If you're going to the doctor's office or the hospital (or you're going somewhere else where you're likely to come in contact with the virus), add a layer of protection by rubbing coconut oil into your skin before you go. Add a few drops of tea tree oil to your coconut oil to enhance the antibacterial effect.

When infections do make their way into the body, coconut oil can help detoxify the body and bolster the immune system. Consuming 3 to 4 teaspoons of coconut oil a day can help the body fight the infection from the inside out. The lauric acid in coconut oil converts to monolaurin once it enters the body. Monolaurin has been shown to be effective against Staphylococcus aureus in laboratory tests.

If you have or suspect you have a staph infection, seek immediate medical advice. Consult with your doctor as to whether you should try using coconut oil to clear the infection up. The stakes are high with certain types of infections and you don't want to try to self-diagnose a staph infection and treat it on your own.

Impetigo

Impetigo is a common skin infection amongst preschool and school-aged children. Symptoms of impetigo include blisters or sores on the extremities and on the neck, head and face. This sort of infection is also common amongst children who wear diapers and have diaper rash or other irritation due to their diapers. Impetigo is typically caused by the staphylococcus aureus bacteria, which we already discussed in the last section, or *streptococcus pyogenes*, which is the bacterium also responsible for causing strep throat.

A child typically gets impetigo when they have another less-serious rash or skin irritation that they scratch or rub repeatedly. The irritation gets infected and blisters or boils start to form.

When there are large blisters in the infected area, the infection is called *bullous impetigo*. If there's small blisters that pop and form into a crust, the infection is called *non-bullous*, or crusted, *impetigo*. The infection tends to be irritated and itchy, which leads the child to scratch it and spread it to other areas of the body. It can also be spread to other children or anyone who comes in contact with the infected area or anything that's touched the infected area.

A combination of coconut oil and tea tree oil can be used as a natural remedy for impetigo. The antibacterial and healing properties of coconut oil and tea tree oil will promote faster healing of impetigo blisters and may help prevent scarring in extreme cases where blisters are prevalent.

As should be the case with any infection, consult with your physician before using coconut oil or tea tree oil.

Folliculitis

Folliculitis is an infection that takes place inside the hair follicles. It can occur anywhere on the body where hair is found, but is most common in the areas of the body where hair is most prevalent, like the face, head and pubic areas. It's typically caused by a bacterial infection, but it can also be caused by fungus or yeast.

Hair follicles that have been irritated by tight clothing or shaving are more prone to developing folliculitis. Those who have other infections, weak immune systems or have been taking antibiotics are also all more susceptible to folliculitis.

Hair follicles with folliculitis are red and irritated and look similar to pimples. They can drain pus and will sometimes have whiteheads. The best way to tell them apart from pimples at a glance is to check and see whether or not there's hair growing from the center. If there are hairs at the center of each inflamed area, chances are it's folliculitis. Your doctor can take samples of the tissue or the fluid leaking from the inflamed area to determine whether it's folliculitis or not.

Mild cases of folliculitis often resolve themselves on their own within a week or two. The healing process can sometimes be sped up a bit by using coconut oil to fight the bacteria or fungus along with the application of warm compresses to help stop the itching and burning. Avoid tight clothing and doing anything that might irritate the infected follicles.

If you have folliculitis and the infection worsens or doesn't get any better, consult with your physician immediately.

Coconut Oil Works on Fungal Infections, Too

People tend to be grossed out when they hear the term "fungal infection" or "yeast infection." The reality is fungi and yeast reside in and on our bodies day in and day out. Fungi thrive in moist areas of the body, like the armpits, the genitals and the areas between the toes. Most these fungi are benign and some can even be beneficial to the body. Others can cause problems, especially if they're allowed to grow unchecked.

Fungal infections can manifest themselves with a number of symptoms. Red, irritated skin, rashes and allergic reactions are all common symptoms. The irritated area isn't always the infected area. At times, allergic reactions to a fungal infection can occur in areas of the body that are distant from the actual area of infection.

There are two basic categories of fungal infection: Yeast infection and dermatophyte infection. *Yeast infections* are commonly caused by *candida albicans yeast*, while *dermatophyte infections* are caused by a variety of different fungi. The good news is coconut oil can often be used as an effective home remedy against both types of fungi.

Foot Fungus

Fungus thrives in moist areas that see little sunlight, so it stands to reason that your feet, which spend long hours sweating enclosed in tight shoes, would harbor large amounts of fungus. Foot fungus is characterized by white lines on the feet and more severe cases result in blistering, cracked skin, itching and burning.

Foot fungus is highly contagious and can be passed from host to host without direct physical contact. Foot fungus is able to live for short periods of time on bathroom floors, in shower stalls and in pools and locker rooms, where it waits for someone to come in contact with it. It can even live in socks and shoes for up to a week. You could be unknowingly reinfecting your feet every time you put on a pair of shoes and your favorite socks.

While not life-threatening, foot fungus can be life-altering, as those who have it are often afraid to show their feet in public. Foot fungus is often associated with being unsanitary, even though it can be contracted by anyone who comes in contact with it.

Foot fungus should be treated at first sign of a fungal infection. If you see the tell-tale white lines of a fungal infection or your feet are starting to crack or itch, it's time to take action. When possible, let your feet air out for long stretches of the day. Change your socks regularly and wait at least a week before wearing the same pair of socks. Wear flip-flops or sandals at the pool and while in locations where reinfection is a risk. Clean and disinfect your bathroom, your shower and other areas your bare feet come in contact with regularly.

Everywhere your bare feet touch is a potential point of reinfection—and an area where others can get infected—so act accordingly. Wear open shoes around the house and apply antifungal powder to your shoes regularly.

Coconut oil is an effective antifungal cream for foot fungus. It can be used on its own or it can be combined with essential oils for topical application only. The following essential oils have antifungal properties and can be combined with coconut oil to combat foot fungus:

- Clove oil.
- Garlic oil.
- Oregano oil.
- Peppermint oil.
- Tea tree oil.

Always dilute essential oils heavily and test new oil blends in a small area before applying it to large areas. Wash and dry your feet before application and leave the oil blend on your feet for as long as possible. Some people report good results when they cover their feet in coconut oil before bedtime and place a plastic bag over their feet to keep the oil from ruining their bedding. They leave the plastic bag on overnight and remove it in the morning, at which time they wash the remaining coconut oil off of their feet and go about their daily business.

Intertrigo

Intertrigo is a skin yeast infection commonly found in the folds of the skin. It's more common in overweight people than it is in thinner people, but it can occur anywhere on the body and can affect anyone. It's most commonly found in fat folds that don't see much sunlight. Women who have had a caesarean section while giving birth sometimes have trouble with intertrigo in and around the flap of skin that can result from the procedure.

Morbidly obese people often suffer from this infection because they have large folds of skin and fat that never see the light of day.

The symptoms of intertrigo are a burning, itching rash, usually found in areas where the skin is folded and dark, moist areas are formed. In addition to being a fungal infection, intertrigo can also be a bacterial infection. Technically, it's any irritation or rash found in the folds of the skin.

Regardless of whether it's fungal or bacterial in nature, Coconut oil can often be used to effectively kill the infection. Mix it with tea tree oil, citronella oil or even patchouli oil for an added boost.

Jock Itch

Jock itch is a fungal infection that occurs in the area of the groin and is characterized by itching and burning of the genitals. Anyone who's suffered jock itch knows it can drive you nuts. You want to scratch yourself in public, but can't out of fear of being seen by someone. Jock itch is caused by a fungus of the name *tinea cruris*, and it primarily affects men. It's common amongst athletes and men who live in warm climates where the genitals are warm and sweaty for most of the day.

Luckily, coconut oil has proven itself an effective remedy for jock itch. It should be applied in the morning before heading out for the day and again in the evening before bed. This is usually enough to put an end to most cases of jock itch, as long as you keep the affected area as clean and dry as possible.

At times, jock itch can come about as a symptom of systemic fungal infection and topical application of coconut oil isn't effective. If jock itch doesn't clear up or symptoms worsen, consult with a physician immediately.

Ringworm

Ringworm is a fungal infection that can be passed from person to person or from animals to people. Contact with an item that has touched an infected person or animal is all that's needed to spread the infection. Swimming pools, showers, locker rooms and contact sports are all ways ringworm is spread.

A ringworm infection is typically characterized by a red, itchy circle on the skin that spreads outward. The skin will feel dry and rough and a ringworm infection can cause bald spots on the scalp. It will spread faster in warm climates than it does when the weather is cold. If you have a burning, itching spot on your skin that turns into a red circle, there's a good chance it's ringworm. Contrary to what many people believe, ringworm doesn't actually involve a worm getting under your skin and digging in. It's a fungal infection that involves fungus getting into the skin. I know that probably still doesn't give you a warm, fuzzy feeling, but at least there isn't a worm crawling around in there.

Coconut oil is a good natural remedy for ringworm infections.

Apply it directly to the infected area at least 3 times a day. The antifungal properties of the oil kill off the fungi and the anti-inflammatory properties help ease the inflammation. Try adding a few drops of lavender or tea tree oil to the coconut oil to further reduce irritation. If this doesn't work, try applying apple cider vinegar to the infected area before using the coconut oil blend. You can also apply coconut oil to a bandage and apply the bandage to the infection, so the coconut oil is present and acting on the infection all day long.

Tinea Versicolor

Tinea versicolor takes place when yeasts that are a normal part of the skin change form into a pathogenic yeast called *Malassezia furfur*. This can occur in anyone, but it's most common in adolescent males, pregnant women, those with suppressed immune systems and people living in tropical climates. A tinea veriscolor infection manifests itself as a raised rash that can either be darker or lighter than the host's skin color.

Since this infection is usually topical, antifungal creams that are rubbed into the skin are a common treatment prescribed by doctors. They work well, but reinfection is common and medications often have to be prescribed more than once to clear up an extensive infection.

Tinea versicolor thrives in oily, moisturized skin, so using moisturizing oils on your skin may actually aid this fungus in taking hold and spreading. Coconut oil is one of the few moisturizing oils that doesn't have this effect because of its natural antifungal properties. Combine a few drops of tea tree oil and lavender oil with your coconut oil before application for an added antifungal effect.

Anti-dandruff shampoos that have antifungal ingredients like selenium sulfide or ketoconazole can also be used on tinea versicolor. They're sold over the counter and can be applied directly to the infection. Lather the shampoo up and let it sit on the infected area for a few minutes before washing it off. These shampoos work well because dandruff is caused by the same fungus that causes tinea versicolor. Once you wash off the shampoo and dry your skin, apply a layer of coconut oil.

Candida Overgrowth

A large number of fungal yeast infections come about as a result of an overgrowth of one particular kind of yeast, *candida albicans*. This harmful yeast is present in all humans in small amounts, but is normally kept in check by beneficial bacteria in the body. When conditions are right, or wrong, as I should say, candida albicans can bloom out of control. This results in what is known as a candida overgrowth.

A *candida overgrowth* is a systemic yeast infection that can cause problems across the entire body. Athlete's foot, jock itch and any number of other skin infections and conditions can come about as a result of a candida overgrowth. In addition to external infections, internal inflammation can occur as the body attempts to fight off the infection. It can manifest itself in all sorts of symptoms, many of which aren't easily linked to a candida overgrowth.

Systemic yeast infections are often misdiagnosed, as doctors diagnose the symptoms and attempt to treat them. The prescribed treatments may work to temporarily rid the body of the symptom, but the infection hasn't been cleared up and symptoms can crop up. The old symptoms can return with a vengeance once treatment is stopped, so if you're having recurring skin yeast infections, a systemic candida overgrowth may be to blame.

Antibiotics prescribed to kill yeast kill beneficial bacteria as well as candida. This leaves plenty of room for Candida to regrow, and grow it often does. Once the good bacteria are gone, there aren't any bacteria left to fight with Candida for space. Antibiotics are largely ineffective against some strains of Candida and can sometimes make things worse.

Studies have shown coconut oil to be an effective tool against drug-resistant Candida. Coconut oil kills Candida albicans yeast. Since an overgrowth is systemic by nature, coconut oil should be taken both externally and orally. Apply it regularly to the infected areas and take 3 to 4 tablespoons of coconut oil a day orally.

Be sure to consult with your doctor prior to using coconut oil as a Candida overgrowth remedy. A rapid die-off of Candida can cause all sorts of new problems to arise and you're going to need to know what to look for.

Dry Skin: Are You Tired of Feeling like a Lizard?

Dry cracked skin can leave you looking and feeling like you belong in the reptile family. A lady I know used to suffer from skin so dry it would crack and bleed. As winter approached, the cool air would cause her dry skin to get even worse and she'd end up with irritated patches of skin that looked and felt like parched leather.

That is, until she discovered coconut oil. She'd heard of it before, but had pretty much given up on getting relief from her dry skin, as she'd tried pretty much every product out there to no avail. Some products would work for a short while, but nothing lasted long enough to provide her any long-term relief.

The first couple days of applying coconut oil were a real eye-opener. She applied it in the morning and again in the evening and watched as her skin became soft and supple and the bloody cracks faded away. She's been using coconut oil for months now and recently told me that her skin has never looked or felt as good as it does now. It definitely looks better, as she doesn't have the visible rough patches she used to have.

Coconut oil helps heal dry, damaged skin and the lipids in the oil penetrate deep to make the skin soft and supple. It has been shown in at least one study to be a better choice for dry skin than mineral oil, which is commonly used as a moisturizer. Simply apply a small amount to the area where the skin is dry and rub it in. If the skin starts feeling dry a little while later, try rubbing in a bit more coconut oil.

There's a fine balance between using the right amount of coconut oil on dry skin and using too much. If you apply too much oil and your skin ends up feeling greasy, rub the oil into other areas of your body. Some people prefer the greasy feeling to having dry skin, but it's a bit much for my tastes. I prefer smaller applications of lesser amounts of oil frequently throughout the day. It leaves my skin feeling soft and supple without leaving me feel like a walking oil slick.

To up the moisturizing effect of coconut oil, try adding equal amounts of cocoa butter and apricot kernel oil to the coconut oil and blending them together.

Psoriasis: Can Coconut Oil Help?

Psoriasis is an autoimmune condition that affects the skin of those who suffer from it. It occurs when the immune system signals the body to start growing skin cells at a faster rate than normal. The most common form of psoriasis is *plaque psoriasis,* which is characterized by raised red patches of skin.

Psoriasis can show up anywhere on the body and anyone can come down with it, although it's more common in people who have compromised immune systems due to other serious health conditions. It is also believed to be caused by stress, food allergies, genetics and a number of other factors.

Outbreaks of psoriasis can range from mild, where only small patches of the body are affected, to severe, where 10 percent or more of the body is covered. If you're suffering an outbreak, it's important to seek medical advice. Certain types of psoriasis can be dangerous and may need immediate medical care.

Coconut oil has seen some use as a natural treatment for the effects of psoriasis.

While it isn't able to completely cure psoriasis, it can ease the effects of the disease and makes life more tolerable for many sufferers. When applied topically, coconut oil is absorbed deep within the skin, where it goes to work knocking out inflammation and aiding with blood flow to the surface capillaries. Users of coconut oil on psoriasis often indicate it doesn't take action immediately. Instead, they notice their symptoms easing up over time.

While there haven't been any notable scientific studies of coconut oil and its effect on psoriasis to date, there is a ton of anecdotal evidence. Forums across the Internet are full of people eschewing coconut oil's virtues when it comes to psoriasis. As with any new treatment, consult with your physician before attempting to use coconut oil to ease the effects of psoriasis.

Sufferers of psoriasis can try adding a few tablespoons of coconut oil a day to their diet as well as applying it topically at least once a day. The anti-inflammatory properties of coconut oil may help fight psoriasis from the inside while bolstering your immune system. It also reduces insulin resistance, which has been linked to psoriasis outbreaks.

Rosacea: Get the Red Out

Rosacea is a chronic skin condition affecting millions of Americans. It's characterized by red, irritated skin, usually on the cheeks and face, but it can also occur on the chest, neck and scalp. Both men and women can have rosacea, but it's much more common in women, especially those of European descent.

Symptoms include redness, irritation, acne, dilated blood vessels near the surface of the skin and red eyes. If you've ever seen an old man or woman with a red, swollen nose, rosacea is more than likely the culprit. If allowed to continue unchecked, it often worsens over time.

The exact cause of rosacea isn't understood. It's an irritation of the skin, but the exact cause of the irritation isn't known. The propensity to suffer rosacea may be at least partially genetic, but scientists don't yet know what touches off an attack. It can come and go, seemingly without warning.

What is known is there are certain triggers that can make rosacea worse. Here are some of the known triggers:

- Anger.
- Certain drugs.
- Drinking.
- Exercise.
- Exertion.
- Extreme hot or cold weather.
- Spicy food.

- Stress.

While none of the above triggers will cause you to develop rosacea if you don't already have it, they can make symptoms worse if you do have it.

There are a number of treatments doctors prescribe for rosacea. If you're suffering a flare-up, contact your doctor for medical advice. Depending on the severity of the attack, your doctor may recommend anything from laser or light therapy to moisturizers and creams. Learning your triggers will allow you to more effectively control your rosacea by avoiding or minimizing triggers.

In addition to prescribed treatments, coconut oil can be applied topically to irritated areas and it can be consumed to fight the inflammation from the inside. Women report that using coconut oil to remove their makeup has helped with redness quite a bit as well.

Milder cases of rosacea can often be controlled by avoiding triggers. Lifestyle adjustments combined with natural remedies like coconut oil may be all a person needs to keep rosacea under control. It's a bad idea to let even mild cases go unchecked, because permanent damage can be done when you allow rosacea flare-ups to persist for long periods of time.

Check with your doctor to see if coconut oil is a good choice for you and apply it to the affected area a couple times a day. If redness persists or gets worse, discontinue use immediately. Coconut oil won't cure rosacea, but it may help ease some of the symptoms and make a flare-up more tolerable.

Help Scars and Stretch Marks Fade Away With Coconut Oil

While they usually aren't painful to the touch or physically irritating, scars and stretch marks can be life-altering, especially if they're located in visible areas. Even when they're covered by clothing, they can still cause angst when it comes time for intimate contact or time to put on a bathing suit and head to the pool.

Coconut oil can work wonders on both scars and stretch marks. It isn't a miracle cure that you rub on and your scars disappear overnight, but it can help fade scars and stretch marks at a much faster pace than they'd normally fade. The best part about using coconut oil is it's entirely natural and doesn't involve harsh chemicals or lasers like some of the other effective scar removal treatments do.

When you apply coconut oil to a scar or stretch mark, it goes to work immediately, penetrating deep within the scar and the skin around it. It protects and heals the skin, and provides nutrients and energy the skin cells need to regenerate. It also softens the skin and makes it more supple, which can help with large areas that have suffered previous damage and are now scarred. While coconut oil probably won't completely eliminate heavy scarring, it may be able to lighten large scars and all but eliminate lighter scars.

Combine coconut oil with vitamin E oil and you've got an even more effective natural treatment for scars. Vitamin

E oil is thought to promote collagen growth and can be key to getting scars to begin healing. Never apply vitamin E oil to open wounds or injuries that haven't finished healing, as it can cause problems. It should only be applied to scars for wounds that have completely healed.

Oil Pulling

Oil pulling is an ancient method of removing toxins from the body. It's easy to do, and the results can be surprising. It doesn't remove toxins from the skin, per se, but instead helps boost the body's immune system. This allows the body to more effectively fight toxins on the skin because it has more resources to throw at them if they attempt to infect the body.

Practicing oil pulling involves taking a teaspoon or two of coconut oil and swishing it around your mouth for 15 to 20 minutes to detoxify your body and pull out all sorts of toxins. Those who swear by it say it helps remove toxins from the entire system, leaving you feeling better.

One of the items oil pulling is said to help with is skin problems.

Whether it works or is just a wives' tale is up for individual interpretation, but I will tell you this. It isn't going to hurt. And it's entirely possible that oil pulling does indeed pull toxins from your body, which in turn helps with healthy skin. It will almost certainly kill bacteria and other microbes that exist in your mouth, which will help ease the load on your body's immune system.

While I can't definitively state that oil pulling works for everyone, there are a lot of people who practice it and swear it works. It's a time-honored practice and it's one that large numbers of people swear by. I do it at least once a week and my skin is healthy, but I also apply coconut oil directly to problem areas, so it's tough to say how much the oil pulling is helping. It has helped whiten my teeth and my chronic halitosis has been all but eliminated, so there's always that.

For best results, try oil pulling in the morning right after you wake up. Never swallow the oil because it's potentially full of toxins you just removed from your body. You don't want to put them right back where they came from. Spit the used oil out into the sink.

Oil pulling can be done with most vegetable oils. Coconut oil is the oil of choice for some people, including myself, because it doesn't have the strong flavor that some other vegetable oils do. Your mileage may vary when it comes to oil pulling. If you're having persistent skin problems and you can't seem to kick them, it's worth at least a shot.

Coconut Oil Homemade Skin Care Product Recipes

There are millions of dollars poured into research and development by the skin care industry and they've yet to come up with a product that's as effective as coconut oil when it comes to leaving the skin feeling happy and healthy. To top things off, coconut oil is less expensive than most skin care products and completely natural. People spend a lot of money for "healthy" skin when many of them would be better off using a natural product like coconut oil as a skin care product.

In addition to using coconut oil on its own, a number of all-natural skin care products can be created using coconut oil as a base or carrier oil. Coconut oil delivers other oils into the skin, penetrating deep below the surface to draw toxins out and carry nutrients in. When you combine coconut oil with other natural ingredients, the skin care possibilities are endless. The recipes in this chapter use all-natural ingredients combined with coconut oil to create healthy all-natural skin care products that are generally much better for you than the products sold commercially.

They're all easy to make and it won't take long to whip up a batch. I don't think there's a single recipe in this section that will take longer than 15 minutes to whip up, regardless of your skill level.

All-Natural Coconut Oil Deodorant

Do a bit of research into what's in the deodorant you've been buying from the store and you'll probably be disgusted by what you've been putting on your skin. Aluminum, formaldehyde and propylene glycol are just a few of the ingredients found in commercial deodorant. Most people think they don't have a choice when it comes to deodorant. It's either use the commercial stuff or smell like body odor.

Try this recipe out and you'll be pleasantly surprised. If you don't like the scent, try playing around with different essential oil blends until you get one you like. The possibilities are unlimited.

Ingredients

½ cup coconut oil

¼ cup baking soda

¼ cup arrowroot powder

1 tablespoon grapefruit juice

5 drops sweet orange essential oil

5 drops tea tree oil

Directions

Combine ingredients together in a glass bowl and blend until incorporated. Store deodorant in a glass container or an empty roll-on deodorant container. Apply it to your armpits in the morning as you would normal deodorant.

Aloe E Sunburn Salve

Coconut oil on its own works great for sunburns. Add vitamin E and aloe vera to the mix and you've got a sunburn salve that eases your pain and helps promote rapid healing.

Ingredients

½ cup coconut oil

½ cup aloe vera gel

6 vitamin E capsules

Directions

Combine the coconut oil and aloe vera gel in a glass bowl and blend together. Poke holes in the vitamin E capsules and pour the contents in the bowl. Mix into the salve. Apply liberally to sunburnt areas at least 3 times a day. If you store this salve for longer than a couple days, you might have to reblend it, as the coconut oil may start to separate from the aloe vera gel.

Antibacterial Hand Sanitizer

Commercial hand sanitizer is made up of mostly alcohol, which can really dry out your skin if you use it often. It also contains a bunch of other chemical compounds you probably shouldn't be applying to your hands on a daily basis.

Ingredients

3 tablespoons coconut oil

1 cup witch hazel

10 drops lavender essential oil

Directions

Add all ingredients to a spray bottle and shake up until mixed. When you want to use the hand sanitizer, shake it up again to mix it and spray it on your hands. You can rub it in. It doesn't have to be washed off.

Antioxidant Passion Fruit Skin Cream

Add papaya and mango to coconut oil and what do you get? A skin cream that smells great and is packed full of antioxidants. This is one of my favorite skin creams because it leaves my skin feeling healthy and elastic, plus I'm a sucker for anything passion fruit.

Ingredients

½ cup coconut oil

1 ripe papaya

1 ripe mango

1 ripe banana

Directions

Add ingredients to a blender and blend until smooth. Rub into skin and let sit for 15 minutes. Wash away and pat dry your skin with a cotton towel. Because of the fresh fruit used in this recipe, it doesn't last long outside of the fridge. It can be stored for a couple days if kept in the fridge.

Sandalwood Antiperspirant

The problem with most homemade deodorants is they don't offer any protection against sweating. They simply prevent you from stinking when you do sweat. This recipe doesn't completely eliminate sweat, but it does a pretty good job of keeping it from reaching the armpits of your clothes. I can't guarantee it'll work for everyone, but it works for my husband, who normally sweats profusely. He applies it a couple times a day and his armpits stay dry all day long.

Be aware that the coconut oil can sometime stain clothing if this antiperspirant is applied in large amounts.

Ingredients

½ cup coconut oil

½ cup aluminum-free baking soda

½ cup corn starch

10 - 15 drops Sandalwood essential oil

Directions

Add all ingredients to a glass mixing bowl and beat until incorporated. Place in the fridge for a few minutes to thicken the mixture up. Spoon the antiperspirant into an old

deodorant container. Store in a cool area. Apply to your
armpits as needed.

Athlete's Foot Salve

Tired of the itching and burning associated with athlete's foot? Whip up a batch of this salve and you'll be able to ease the irritation while helping clear up the infection. This all-natural salve also works well to eliminate foot odor due to fungal infections.

Ingredients

½ cup coconut oil

1 teaspoon neem oil

1 teaspoon baking soda

½ teaspoon grapefruit juice

4 drops tea tree oil

Directions

Mix ingredients together and store in a glass container. When athlete's foot or foot fungus flares up apply this salve liberally and leave on as long as possible. Apply daily until infection has been gone for at least 5 days.

Oatmeal Yogurt Inflammation Busting Cream

Need a soothing cream for itchy, irritated skin? The oatmeal, yogurt and aloe vera in this cream combine with the coconut oil and coconut cream to create a soothing salve that'll knock down inflammation in no time at all.

Ingredients

¼ cup coconut oil

¼ cup coconut cream

¼ cup aloe vera gel

1 tablespoon oatmeal powder

2 tablespoons plain yogurt

Directions

Combine all ingredients and stir together. If you don't have oatmeal powder, you can make it by blending regular oatmeal in a blender or a food processor. Place the mixture in the fridge to cool before use. Apply it to your skin and gently rub it in. Let sit for 15 to 30 minutes and gently wash off. Pat your face dry with a cotton towel.

Oily Skin Face Wash

This face wash contains lemon juice, which has astringent properties, so it works well for people with oily skin. Instead of lemon juice, you can substitute a few drops of lemon essential oil, if your skin can handle it. Either way, oily skin will soon be a thing of the past.

Ingredients

½ cup coconut oil

5 drops tea tree oil

5 drops lavender oil

1 tablespoon lemon juice

Directions

Add ingredients to a glass bowl and blend until incorporated. To use, apply to your face and leave on for a few minutes and then wash away.

Shea Butter Shaving Cream

This homemade shaving cream is a rich blend of butters and oils that go on easy and leave the skin you're shaving smelling good and feeling smooth. It works well for difficult to shave areas with thick hair.

Ingredients

½ cup coconut oil

½ cup Shea butter

¼ cup almond oil

OPTIONAL: 5 to 10 drops of your favorite essential oil

Directions

Melt the coconut oil and Shea butter in a saucepan over low heat. Stir in the almond oil. Remove the saucepan from the heat and stir in 5 to 10 drops of your favorite essential oil or oil blend, if so desired. When the oil blend thickens up, beat it with a blender until it's thick and frothy.

Use it the same way you would any other shaving cream.

Smooth Skin Serum

Blend coconut oil with other plant oils and an essential oil or two and you get a serum that leaves your skin feeling nourished and hydrated. All it takes is a few drops a day to leave dry, damaged skin feeling nice and smooth.

<u>Ingredients</u>

½ cup coconut oil

3 tablespoons almond oil

3 tablespoons sweet apricot oil

3 drops avocado oil

3 to 5 drops carrot seed oil

<u>Directions</u>

Combine all of the oils in a glass container and stir until completely blended. Apply a few drops daily of this serum to skin you want to nourish and moisturize and rub it in. You'll have happy, healthy skin year-round.

Ultimate Skin Tonic

Use this all-purpose tonic on your skin year-round to leave it feeling smooth, silky and healthy. It moisturizes the skin and feeds it plenty of nutrients, leaving you feeling pampered and clean. You could spend a lot of money on expensive creams and tonics, but there's no need to when you have this lotion!

Ingredients

½ cup coconut oil

¼ cup rosehip seed oil

2 tablespoons extra virgin olive oil

2 tablespoons jojoba oil

10 drops frankincense essential oil

Directions

Add all of the ingredients to a glass bowl and blend until completely incorporated. Apply to your skin daily or on an as-needed basis.

Vanilla Lavender Lip Balm

If you're anything like me, you get chapped lips in both the summer and the winter. And if you're like me, you've struggled to find a good all-natural lip balm that doesn't break the bank.

Chances are, you'll love this lip balm, both for summer and winter application. It's good stuff and it smells fantastic. If you don't care for the lavender smell, and I know there's a few of you who don't, leave it out. You can replace it with an essential oil you do like or just go with the vanilla scent. Your call.

Ingredients

¼ cup coconut oil

¼ cup Shea butter

¼ cup beeswax

10 drops vanilla essential oil

10 drops lavender essential oil

Directions

Melt the coconut oil, Shea butter and beeswax in a saucepan over low heat. Stir together and remove from heat. Let it cool a bit and stir in the lavender and vanilla oil before it solidifies. Divide into personal containers that you can carry with you. Apply whenever your lips start to feel a little chapped.

Super-Creamy Whipped Peppermint Body Butter

One of my biggest complaints about coconut oil used to be the fact that when it got cold in the house, my jar of coconut oil turned into a solid and it was difficult to get the oil out of the jar. Whipping coconut oil together with Shea butter and vitamin E oil creates a creamy lotion that doesn't harden up when it gets cold in the house.

This is a great lotion to have on hand in the winter because it soothes wind- and cold-burnt skin. Be aware that peppermint oil can be "hot" and may irritate the skin. Test this butter in small amounts before applying it to a larger area.

Ingredients

½ cup coconut oil

½ cup Shea butter

1 teaspoon vitamin E oil

3 to 5 drops peppermint essential oil

Directions

Add all ingredients to a mixing bowl. The coconut oil and Shea butter must be solid in order for the whipping process to work. Mix with a mixer on High speed using a wire whisk attachment for 5 to 10 minutes. The butter is done when it has been whipped into a light, frothy consistency. Store in a cool area where the butter will remain solid. If your house is too warm, store the butter in the fridge.

Moisturizing Shaving Lotion

This simple to make shaving lotion is gentle enough to be used on your legs. It can also be used for shaving whiskers and other areas with thick hair. It does a good job of lubricating the skin and it moisturizes while you shave. The tea tree oil helps reduce the chance of razor burn and further conditions the skin.

Ingredients

½ cup coconut oil

5 to 10 drops tea tree oil

Directions

Blend the coconut oil and tea tree oil together in a glass container. Apply liberally to the area you plan on shaving. Shave and then reapply as an aftershave lotion if necessary.

Avocado Coconut Face Mask

This mask combines the moisturizing effect of avocado with that of coconut oil. It works well for most skin types and is great for damaged and dry skin.

Ingredients

½ cup coconut oil

2 teaspoons avocado oil

½ ripe avocado, mashed

3 tablespoons honey

Directions

Combine ingredients in a glass bowl and blend together until incorporated. Apply mask to face and leave on for 30 minutes. Wash the mask off and pat your face dry.

Because this mask uses fresh avocado, it has to be stored in the fridge in an airtight container. It will only last a few days, so be sure to use it quickly.

Banana Coconut Anti-Aging Face Mask

Bananas are rich in vitamins and work well when used in anti-aging creams. Combining bananas and coconut oil can work wonders for your skin, leaving your skin feeling fresh and rejuvenated.

Ingredients

½ cup coconut oil

1 ripe banana

¼ cup honey

Directions

Mash banana until smooth and creamy. Add all ingredients to a glass bowl and mix until incorporated. Apply mask to face and leave on for 20 to 30 minutes. Wash face and pat dry with a soft towel.

Because this mask uses fresh banana, it has to be stored in the fridge in an airtight container. It will only last a day or two, so be sure to use it quickly.

Coconut Oil Exfoliating Scrub

This recipe is designed to moisturize the skin and to exfoliate away dead skin cells. The coconut oil moisturizes the skin and provides it with nutrients while the brown sugar and sea salt lift away dead skin cells and the toxins drawn out by the oil.

Ingredients

½ cup coconut oil

3 tablespoons brown sugar

¼ cup honey

¼ cup sea salt

Directions

Combine ingredients in a glass bowl and blend together. The ingredients should be thoroughly mixed, but not blended so much the salt and sugar is incorporated into the oil. The crystals have to be somewhat intact to exfoliate the skin.

To use the exfoliating scrub, apply it to your skin and gently rub it into your skin in a circular motion. Let it sit for 5 to 10 minutes and wash it off.

Diaper Rash Cream

While you're making all-natural products for yourself, you might as well go ahead and whip up a batch of this diaper rash cream for your little guy or gal. The zinc oxide is optional. Some people prefer to use it, while others prefer to stick with more natural items for their cream.

If you do decide to use zinc oxide, be aware that this diaper cream may not be cloth diaper safe. I've heard of people using it in small amounts with no issues, but don't recommend it.

Ingredients

½ cup coconut oil

1 cup Shea butter

3 tablespoons vegetable glycerin

2 tablespoons beeswax

OPTIONAL: 1 tablespoon zinc oxide

Directions

Melt the coconut butter and Shea butter over low heat. Add the beeswax and stir until blended. Remove from heat and let the mixture start to cool. Add the vegetable glycerin (and the zinc oxide, if you want to use it) and stir it in. Let the cream solidify and beat until creamy.

When you want to use it, apply a small amount to the area where the diaper rash is present.

Extra Hydration Face Mask

Are you plagued with excessively dry skin? This face mask provides extra hydration and will leave your skin feeling hydrated and smooth.

Ingredients

½ cup coconut oil

2 tablespoons honey

1 ripe avocado, mashed

2 tablespoons powdered milk

3 to 5 drops evening primrose oil

Directions

Mash the avocado and combine all ingredients in a glass bowl. Combine until incorporated. Apply to face and leave on skin for 10 to 15 minutes. Wash off and pat dry with cotton towel.

Because this mask uses fresh avocado, it has to be stored in the fridge in an airtight container. It will only last a few days, so be sure to use it quickly.

Eye Makeup Remover

Are you looking for a makeup remover that softens the skin as it gently removes makeup? This non-toxic makeup remover fits the bill. Use it on sensitive areas and watch as the makeup just wipes away.

Ingredients

½ cup extra virgin olive oil

½ cup coconut oil

Directions

Blend the two oils together in a glass jar. To remove makeup, dip a cotton ball in the makeup remover and use it to wipe away the makeup. It should wipe right off. If not, try applying the remover to your makeup and let it sit for 30 seconds. Wipe the makeup away using a soft towel.

Eye Cream

Here's an all-natural eye cream that will help fight the effects of aging. The coconut oil helps reduce and repair wrinkles at the corners of your eyes, while the vitamin E has antioxidant and anti-aging qualities.

Ingredients

½ cup coconut oil

5 capsules vitamin E oil

Directions

Melt the coconut oil in a saucepan over low heat. Poke holes in the vitamin E capsules and pour the contents into the melted coconut oil. Stir the vitamin E into the coconut oil. Let the mixture cool and harden. You can speed the process up by putting it in the fridge. Whip the mixture until light and creamy.

Apply to the skin around your eyes, being careful not to get the eye cream in your eyes. This cream can also be applied to other problem areas to help smooth out wrinkles.

Coconut Oil Bug Repellent

Rather than spraying yourself with toxic chemicals like DEET, you can use this coconut oil-based insect repellent to repel insects naturally. While some bug repellent recipes call for citrus oils, be aware that citrus essential oils can be phototoxic, meaning they cause a reaction with your skin when exposed to sunlight. This repellent doesn't use any citrus oils. You can add citrus oils if you like, just be sure to apply the repellent to areas that aren't exposed to the sun.

Ingredients

½ cup coconut oil

¼ cup Shea butter

3 tablespoons beeswax

5 drops NEEM oil

10 drops citronella essential oil

10 drops Cedarwood essential oil

10 drops eucalyptus essential oil

Directions

Melt coconut oil, Shea butter and beeswax in a saucepan over low heat. You can use a double broiler if you have one. Stir the oils and the wax together until they're blended.

Remove from heat and add the essential oils. Stir them in until incorporated. Let cool and store in a glass container.

Be careful when you use this bug repellent because it contains a lot of essential oils. Always test it on a small area prior to application. This repellent may not last all day. If it loses effectiveness, reapply it as needed.

Lavender Coconut Face Wash

This face wash features lavender essential oil, which gives it a soothing and interesting scent and ups the antibacterial qualities of the face wash. It's great for dry, irritated skin because it eases inflammation and moisturizes the skin.

Ingredients

½ cup coconut oil

5 to 10 drops lavender essential oil

¼ cup honey

Directions

Combine ingredients in a glass bowl and stir together until incorporated. Add lavender essential oil a drop or two at a time and stir in until desired aroma is reached.

Apply to face and leave on for a couple minutes. Wash it off and pat your face dry with a towel.

Lemon Sugar Scrub

I'm a big fan of this sweet and sour sugar scrub. The sugar exfoliates the skin and the lemon juice tightens up the pores. The coconut oil . . . Well, you know what it does.

Ingredients

½ cup coconut oil

2 cups table sugar

2 cups lemon juice

Directions

Combine the table sugar and coconut oil and stir together. Slowly add lemon juice and stir it in until a thick paste is formed. You can use it to scrub and exfoliated the skin on your body and on your face. Simply rub it on in a circular motion and wash it away.

Lemon Whipped Body Butter

I love lemon scented products. I clean my house with all-natural lemon scented products and I love to use them for skin care as well. This lemon body butter reminds me of lemon crème pie. It smells great and leaves my skin feeling great as well. I hope you love it as much as I do.

Ingredients

1 cup coconut oil

2 tablespoons castor oil

1 teaspoon vitamin E oil

1 tablespoon aloe vera gel

15 drops lemon essential oil

Directions

Add all of the ingredients to a mixing bowl. Make sure the coconut oil is in solid form. Use a wire whisk attachment on an electric mixer to whip the ingredients until they are completely incorporated and the butter is a light, creamy consistency. This usually takes around 5 minutes, but can take a bit longer.

Store your butter in a cool location where it won't melt. If it melts, it will lose its consistency. If you live in a warm climate, the butter can be stored in the fridge.

Use as needed by applying the butter to your skin and rubbing it in.

The Human Hair: What You Need to Know

Hair is found all over the human body, but most people know surprisingly little about the anatomy of their hair and the follicles their hair grows from. If you already know everything there is to know about your hair, you can skip this chapter. If not, there's a lot of good information here that'll help you understand your hair and why you might be having certain problems with it.

Hair grows from structures in the skin known as *hair follicles*. There are millions of follicles on the body and each follicle grows a single hair made of a protein called *keratin*. You are born with the maximum number of follicles you're going to have. The human body doesn't produce any hair follicles after birth.

At the base of each follicle lies the *hair bulb*, which is the area of the follicle that produces the cells that make up the hair. Cells grow and divide in the bulb and are slowly pushed out of the follicle as growth occurs. As the cells leave the hair bulb, they die and form into the shaft of the hair. The *sebaceous gland* produces *sebum*, which is an oil that lubricates the hair and naturally conditions the hair and surrounding skin. If you have oily hair and skin, excess sebum production is likely the culprit.

There are three phases in the hair growth cycle. The *anagen phase* is the growth phase. This is the phase in which hair grows and is pushed out of the follicle. This is the longest phase of the hair growth cycle and can last for years. The anagen phase lasts for a set amount of time. This means each strand of hair will only grow to a certain length. If you have hair that undergoes a naturally short anagen phase, your hair won't grow long no matter what you do. This is the reason why some people are able to grow really long hair, while others can try forever to let their hair grow out and it never passes a certain length.

The *catagen phase* is the phase during which the hair follicle transitions from growing hair to being dormant. The follicle shrinks and the growth of the hair slows to a crawl. This phase lasts anywhere from a couple weeks to month.

In the resting phase, or the *telogen phase*, hair follicles shed the hair they've been growing and go dormant for a couple months while they rest and prepare to restart the cycle. Eventually, the anagen phase starts again and the cycle starts over.

At any given time, you have hair follicles on your head in all of the three states. Each follicle is on its own growth cycle. If all of the follicles were on the same cycle, your hair would grow to a certain length and then all fall out at once. Luckily this isn't the case. Each individual follicle is on its own cycle, albeit one that can be modified by hormonal signals sent by the brain.

The shaft of the hair consists of three layers. The *medulla* is the innermost layer. The size of the medulla varies from person to person and from hair shaft to hair shaft, even on the same person. Some hair doesn't have a medulla at all.

The *cortex* is the next layer. It's sandwiched between the cuticle, which is the outer layer of the hair, and the medulla. The cortex is the thickest part of the hair, often making up as much as 90% of the weight of a strand of hair. It's made up of strands of keratin and protein that determine the hair's elasticity and volume.

The outer layer of the hair is called the *cuticle*. It's made up of interlocked scales that lock tightly together in healthy hair to protect the inside layers of the hair. When you think of the cuticle layer, think of shingles on a roof. As the hair gets damaged, the shingles lift and it becomes harder to keep the hair hydrated and healthy. Dying the hair creates breaks in the cuticle layer because the dye has to get into the shaft in order to effectively color the hair. Healthy hair shines because the cuticle layer is locked together tightly to create a smooth surface. Damaged hair is often dull because many of the cuticle scales are lifted and don't have the same reflective properties.

When the cuticle layer becomes badly damaged, hair has trouble holding moisture and it begins to lose protein. It becomes dry and brittle and is prone to split ends and breakage. The more damaged it gets, the more unmanageable it becomes. Damaged hair soaks up moisture when it's washed, causing the hair to swell. The moisture then leaks out quickly, causing the hair to shrink. The rapid expansion and shrinkage of the hair during washing does even more damage to the cuticle layer.

When a person has damaged hair that's difficult to manage, the typical response is to use more heat and more product to hold the hair in place. This creates a vicious cycle in which the hair becomes even more damaged as the person has to do more and more to it to get it styled. It eventually succumbs to the cumulative damage and breaks off.

If you've got brittle or thin hair that's prone to breakage and you've been using a lot of products and/or heat on your hair, it's time to break the cycle. Stop heating your hair and using dyes and other products on it for a while and give new, undamaged hair a chance to grow out. This is the best way to heal your hair, as badly damaged hair isn't repairable. You can mask the damage with products like coconut oil, but continuing to use heat and styling products with coconut oil will continue the cycle.

How Coconut Oil Helps the Hair

Coconut oil goes a long way toward stopping the cycle of damage done to your hair by repeated use of heat and styling products. While it doesn't reverse the damage that's already been done, it does a great job of masking the damage while protecting the hair from further damage. Coconut oil is one of the best products for conditioning the hair and protecting the hair from damage because it acts on the hair in multiple beneficial ways.

It works best as a pre-wash treatment, used in the hair before you wash it with your normal shampoo and conditioner. This is because coconut oil works its way deep into the shaft of the hair. It doesn't just coat the cuticle, it actually works itself into the cortex, where it takes hold and repels water from making its way into the shaft. It effectively seals damaged hair from taking up water, protecting it from the swelling that would otherwise take place.

The fatty acids in coconut oil have a high affinity for the proteins found in hair. This helps the coconut oil to penetrate deeper into the shaft than other oils because the hair protein draws it in. Once inside, it holds the protein in place and helps prevent protein loss when the hair is washed.

The more damaged or porous your hair is, the more it can benefit from having coconut oil applied to it. Badly damaged hair and porous hair types like natural hair will benefit most, but coconut oil can be used on all hair types. In addition to locking moisture out and protein in, coconut oil also coats the outside of the hair, making it more supple and workable. When hair is damaged the raised cuticles catch on one another as hair slides across itself. Coconut oil lubricates the hair, allowing it to slide smoothly without catching.

This prevents further damage and allows you to easily brush and style your hair.

It's important to remember that coconut oil isn't actually repairing the damage to your hair. The effects of using coconut oil are temporary and damaged hair will eventually return to its damaged state. Coconut oil and coconut oil products can be reapplied when hair again becomes unruly, but it won't work miracles and restore damaged hair to a healthy state. The only way to do that is to grow out new hair that hasn't endured years of abuse.

Coconut oil can help bridge the gap and extend the life of damaged hair until new hair can be grown out. Stop the abuse now before it's too late.

Coconut Oil and Head Lice

By now, you've got to be wondering if there's anything coconut oil can't do. Well, here's another thing it can do: fight lice. Studies have shown coconut oil to be an effective all-natural treatment for head lice.

Yeah, I was pretty excited when I found this out, too. If you have kids, you've probably already battled head lice a time or two. If not, there's a pretty good chance your children aren't going to make it through their school years completely unscathed. People tend to associate head lice with unsanitary conditions, but the truth is it doesn't matter how clean you keep your home (or your kids). All it takes is brushing up against someone or something with head lice on it, like another kid or a jacket, and you've got an infestation to deal with.

If you're lucky, you catch it early, before the lice have populated your house and infected everyone in the house. If you're unlucky, you have to treat everyone in your house and you have to take steps to eliminate the lice from the house itself.

The normal course of treatment for head lice involves running out to the local drug store or pharmacy and paying an arm and a leg for expensive lice shampoo. This shampoo works well, but is packed full of chemicals that are readily absorbed by the scalp of those to which it's applied. You're killing the lice, but at what cost? Who knows what long-term damage is being done to the system of those who the shampoo has been applied to. For many years, people have accepted these toxic shampoos as their only course of head lice treatment.

I'm not sure who the first person to try coconut oil as a head lice remedy was but whoever it is, I owe them a huge hug. Now, instead of sitting at home sucking in toxic fumes every time my kids are infested, I can treat them with coconut oil. It's good for their hair, their scalp and my sanity, as it's an effective treatment that more often than not knocks out lice the first time I apply it.

Here are the steps you need to take to clear up lice using coconut oil:

1. **Massage enough coconut oil into the hair to coat the hair.**
2. **Comb through the hair with a nit comb.** Go section by section and be sure to remove every visible nit. Start at the base of each section of hair and comb all the way to the end.
3. **Apply liberal amounts of coconut oil to the hair.** Be sure to massage it throughout the hair and deep into the scalp.
4. **Cover the hair with a shower cap and leave the coconut oil in the hair for at least 6 hours and preferably 12.**
5. **Wash the coconut oil out of the hair.**
6. **Repeat the combing process to remove any remaining nits.**
7. **If necessary, repeat the process a week or two later to get rid of any stragglers that may have made it through the initial treatment.**

You have to make sure you disinfect your house and get rid of any lice that may be in your clothes, furniture and your carpet. If not, you're going to end up with an infestation that continuously reinfects your family, no matter what you do. If you keep finding new lice in your family's hair, you probably haven't done enough to get rid of the lice in your house.

The good news is lice in the home are fairly easy to eradicate. Wash all laundry with hot water and seal items that have touched the head that can't be washed in a plastic bag for at least a week. Most lice will die off within a day or two if they don't have a host to feed on. Fumigant sprays aren't usually necessary, which is good because they're packed full of toxic chemicals.

Coconut Oil Hair Care Recipes

Coconut oil is great for your hair on its own, but it's even better when combined with other all-natural ingredients. Coconut oil hair care products can be used to replace most of the harsh chemical products you're used to using. Instead of continuing to damage your hair with chemical products that mask problems while doing nothing to prevent them, it's time to switch over to natural products that are easy on your hair. Instead of covering up problems while potentially creating new ones, coconut oil is easy enough on your hair that it will allow it time to regrow.

While there aren't any products that will completely repair damaged hair, coconut oil is as close as it gets because it gets inside the shaft and helps the hair maintain its integrity. Start using coconut oil today and you'll see an almost immediate difference.

The hair care product recipes in this chapter feature coconut oil as one of their main ingredients. If you're using chemical hair care products, it's time to consider making the switch to coconut oil. Feel free to play around with the amount of coconut oil used in these recipes. Certain hair types will feel heavier than others when coconut oil is used, so if you aren't happy, add or remove coconut oil until you've fine-tuned the recipe to your liking.

All-Natural Styling Gel

Looking for a natural styling gel? This gel doesn't quite lock your hair in place like commercial gel, but it's a passable (and all-natural) alternative. Try it out and see if you like it.

Ingredients

½ cup coconut oil

½ cup mango butter

¼ cup Shea butter

½ cup aloe vera gel

1 tablespoon vegetable glycerin

Directions

Melt the coconut oil, mango butter and the aloe vera gel. Add the rest of the ingredients and stir them in. Remove from heat and let solidify before use. If this recipe doesn't have enough holding power, try adding a bit of beeswax.

Brittle Hair Treatment

Damaged or thin hair can be extremely brittle. If you have hair that easily breaks when you comb or brush it or you're constantly finding a bunch of broken off strands of hair on your pillow, this treatment may shore the strength up a bit, making your hair more manageable.

Ingredients

½ cup coconut oil

1 ripe avocado, mashed

2 tablespoons honey

Directions

Add all ingredients to a mixing bowl and blend together. You'll end up with a green-tinted creamy paste. Apply it to your hair and cover your hair with a shower cap. Let it sit for 30 minutes to half an hour and then rinse it out. Condition your hair like you normally would.

This recipe has to be stored in the fridge. It'll only last a few days, so be sure to use it up before them.

Coconut Almond Conditioner

This conditioner gets deep inside your hair and seals moisture in. It nourishes your hair and smooths out the cuticles. The best part is it's all-natural, so you can use it as often as you need to.

<u>Ingredients</u>

½ cup coconut oil

¼ cup almond oil

1 teaspoon vitamin E oil

<u>Directions</u>

Combine ingredients and blend together. Apply to hair and let sit for 30 minutes to an hour. Completely wash the conditioner out and your hair will be supple and workable.

Coconut Lavender Conditioner

If you love the smell of lavender, you'll love this conditioner. If not, well, what the heck is wrong with you? Just kidding . . . but seriously, this is a great conditioner. If you really don't care for the lavender oil, try substituting another essential oil that you do like.

Ingredients

½ cup coconut oil

¼ cup water

¼ cup Grapeseed oil

1 teaspoon vitamin E oil

15 drops lavender essential oil

Directions

Heat the cup of water in the microwave for a minute or two, until it's warm enough to melt the coconut oil in. Add the coconut oil and stir it in. Add the rest of the ingredients and stir them until incorporated. To use, work small amounts of the conditioner into your hair. Leave it in for 15 to 20 minutes and wash out.

If you let this conditioner sit for more than a day or two, the oil and water will start to separate. Shake it up before using it to recombine the oil and water. If you want a thicker conditioner, you can leave out the water.

Dry Hair Treatment

This treatment adds moisture to your hair and locks it in. What more could you ask of a dry hair treatment?

Ingredients

½ cup coconut oil

¼ cup mayonnaise

1 ripe avocado

1 ripe banana

Directions

Mash the banana and avocado. Combine all of the ingredients in a mixing bowl and blend together. Apply liberally to your hair and cover it with a shower cap. Let sit for 45 minutes and then completely wash out.

Because of the avocado and banana, this treatment doesn't store very well. Keep it in the fridge and use within a day or two for best results.

Dull Hair Treatment

Is your hair losing its lustrous shine? Use this dull hair treatment to restore your hair's natural shine. This treatment improves shine and improves the overall health of your hair. Apply it at least once a week for best results.

Ingredients

½ cup coconut oil

2 tablespoons almond oil

2 tablespoons extra virgin olive oil

3 tablespoons ground dried hibiscus flowers

Directions

Combine all of the ingredients in a mixing bowl and whisk together until thoroughly mixed. To treat your hair, apply it to your hair and massage the treatment into your hair and scalp. Wrap your head in a warm towel and leave the treatment in for 45 minutes. Wash it out and wash and condition your hair as you normally would.

Herbal Color Enhancer

If the color of your hair is fading, you can use this color enhancer to rejuvenate your hair. The parsley added to this recipe will make your hair radiant and it should make the color really pop.

Ingredients

½ cup coconut oil

2 tablespoons ground parsley

2 tablespoons sage

1 teaspoon vitamin E oil

Directions

Add the ingredients to a mixing bowl and blend until rich and creamy. To use, apply the color enhancer to your hair and leave it in for a couple hours. Place a shower cap over your head to keep the coconut oil on your hair where it belongs.

Moisturizing Curl Spray

Use this spray to give naturally curly hair a boost any time you need it. It uses the moisturizing properties of aloe vera combined with a bit of coconut oil to create the perfect curl spray. Don't go too heavy on the coconut oil in this spray or it will leave your curls looking oily and matted.

Ingredients

1 cup distilled water

¼ cup aloe vera juice

3 tablespoons coconut oil

Directions

Melt the coconut oil. Add the coconut oil and the rest of the ingredients to a spray bottle and shake until combined. Whenever your curls start to look flat, give them a light misting of this spray.

Overnight Hair Mask

This hair mask is designed to be added to your hair in the evening before you go to bed and left in your hair all night. It'll leave your hair feeling amazing, especially if you suffer from dry or brittle hair.

Ingredients

½ cup coconut oil

½ cup Shea butter

¼ cup almond oil

¼ cup jojoba oil

3 teaspoons vitamin E oil

Directions

Melt butters and oils together in a saucepan over low heat. Remove from heat and stir in the vitamin E oil. Coat your hair with this mask in the evening and cover your hair with a shower cap. You might also want to cover your pillow with a thick towel to catch any leakage. In the morning, wash the hair mask completely out of your hair.

Scalp Salve

Your hair isn't the only thing taking a beating when you use chemical-laden products. Your scalp gets beat up, too.

This scalp salve combines the soothing effects of tea tree oil and peppermint oil to create a salve that leaves your scalp feeling clean and fresh instead of dry and itchy.

Ingredients

½ cup coconut oil

½ cup Shea butter

½ cup aloe vera juice

5 to 10 drops peppermint oil

5 to 10 drops tea tree oil

Directions

Melt the coconut oil and Shea butter in a saucepan over low heat. Add the aloe vera juice and stir it in. Remove from heat and let the salve cool until it starts to thicken. Stir in the essential oils. To use, apply the salve directly to the scalp and massage it in.

Be aware that this combination of essential oils may be a dermal irritant for some. Always test in small amounts in an inconspicuous area before applying the salve to a larger area.

Vanilla Coconut Milk Shampoo

There are numerous chemicals in commercial shampoo that don't belong anywhere near your head. You use it on your hair, but when you rinse it out, it gets on your scalp and runs down your body. Exactly how much of the chemicals you absorb into your body isn't clear, but one thing's for certain. You won't absorb any of the chemicals if you switch over to a natural alternative.

Ingredients

½ cup coconut milk

½ cup liquid castile soap

2 tablespoons coconut oil

1 teaspoon vitamin E oil

5 to 10 drops vanilla essential oil

Directions

Combine all ingredients in a bottle and shake until they're thoroughly mixed. Give them a good shake before using the shampoo because the oil will separate from the soap. To use, massage a dab of the shampoo into your hair and wash it out.

Other Books You May Be Interested In

Many of the recipes in this book use essential oils. If you want more information on essential oils and their applications, I recommend the following book:

The Aromatherapy & Essential Oils Handbook

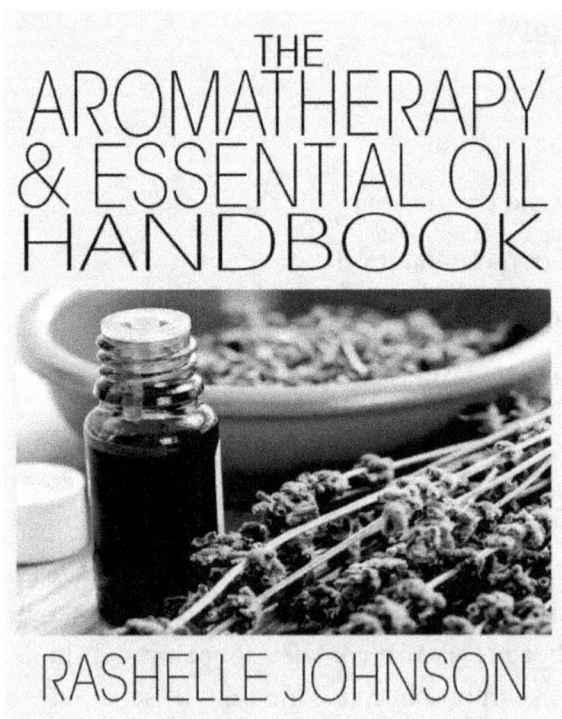

http://www.amazon.com/dp/B00BECCJXY

Diet plays a huge role in healthy skin. If you're interested in healthy eating, there are a number of healthy foods you may be interested in adding to your diet. The following books may be of interest to you.

The Coconut Flour Cookbook: Delicious Gluten Free Coconut Flour Recipes

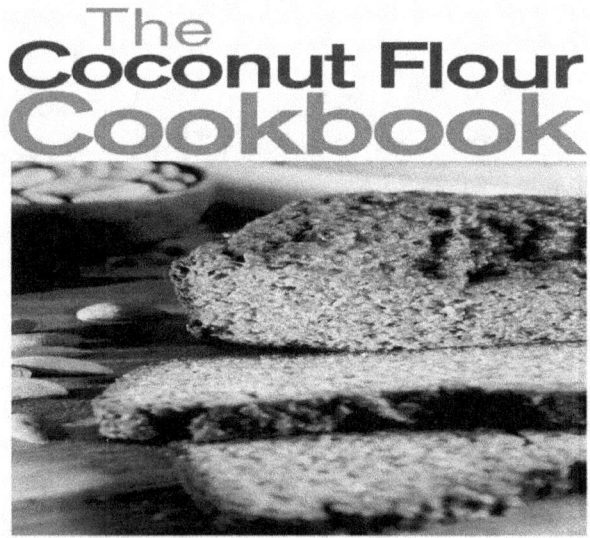

http://www.amazon.com/dp/B00CC0JFPM

The Almond Flour Cookbook: 30 Delicious and Gluten Free Recipes

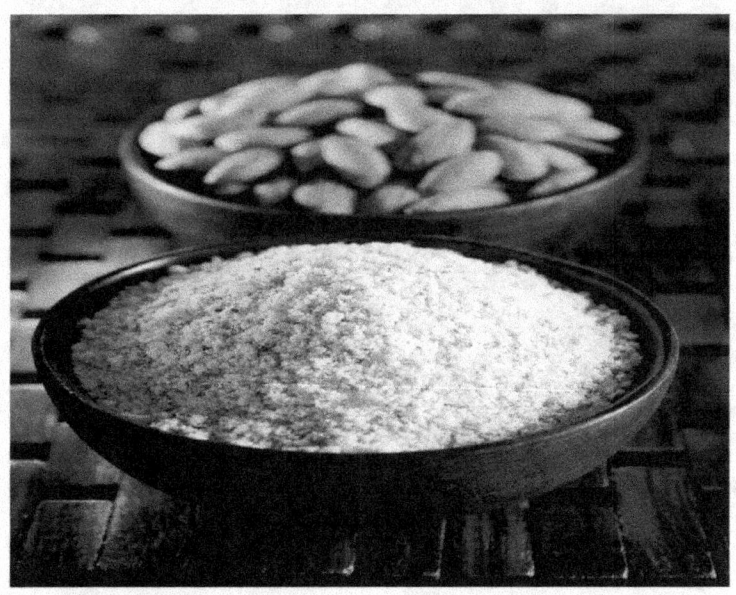

http://www.amazon.com/dp/B00CB3SJ0M

The Quinoa Cookbook: Healthy and Delicious Quinoa Recipes (Superfood Cookbooks)

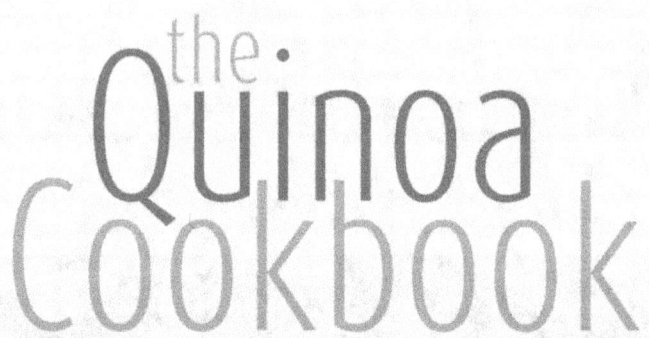

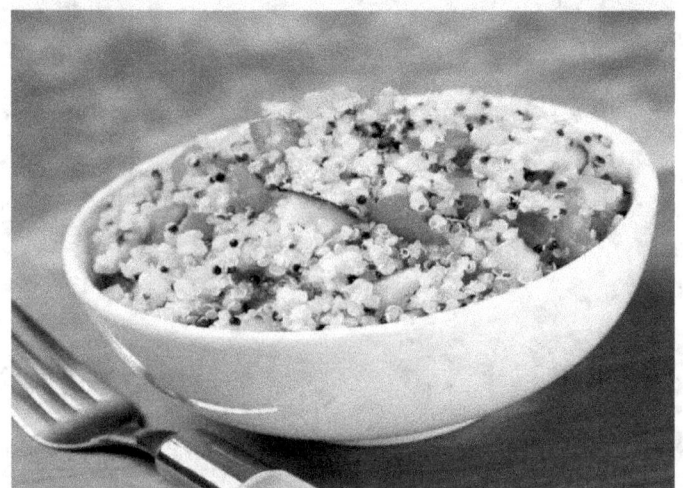

http://www.amazon.com/dp/B00B2T2420

www.ingramcontent.com/pod-product-compliance
Lightning Source LLC
Chambersburg PA
CBHW070705290526
45790CB00001B/462